Diverticulitis Meal Prep For Beginners

Nutritious Recipes for a Healthy Digestive System and Ready-to-go Meals to Prevent Painful Flare-ups

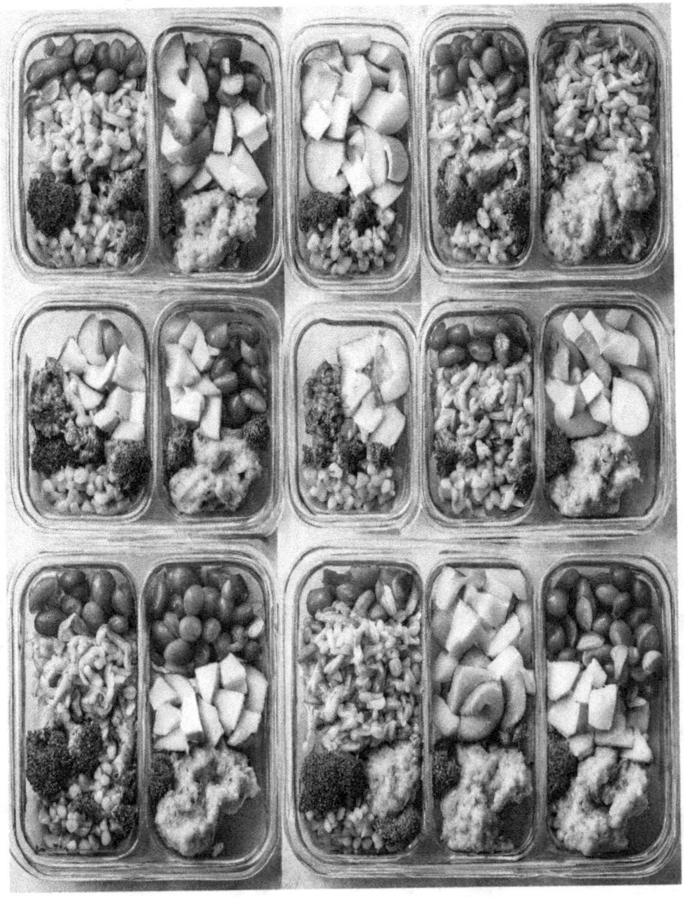

Dr. Tate Mandara

Table of Contents

INTRODUCTION

Roland, a vibrant and determined retiree, was no stranger to the challenges posed by diverticulitis. Frequent bouts of abdominal pain and digestive discomfort had become a part of his daily life. It was frustrating, to say the least, for someone who had always been active and enjoyed preparing meals from scratch. One day, as he was browsing the internet for solutions, Roland stumbled upon the concept of meal prepping for diverticulitis. The idea of planning and preparing meals ahead of time piqued his interest, and he decided to give it a try.

He began by researching diverticulitis-friendly recipes and creating a weekly meal plan. Roland meticulously washed and chopped vegetables, cooked grains, and portioned out lean proteins.

He discovered a variety of dishes that suited his condition, from hearty quinoa salads to soothing soups and stews, all loaded with fiber and low on irritants. As weeks passed, Roland realized that his new meal-prepping routine was making a remarkable difference. The pre-planned meals allowed him to control portion sizes and incorporate the right ingredients while avoiding trigger foods. The abdominal pain lessened, and his digestion improved.

With his newfound freedom from constant pain, Roland rekindled his passion for gardening and leisurely strolls. Meal prepping had become his ally in the battle against diverticulitis, giving him not only better health but also the joy of a more active life.

CHAPTER ONE

UNDERSTANDING DIVERTICULITIS

What Is Diverticulitis?

Diverticulitis is a digestive disorder characterized by inflamed or infected pouches (diverticula) in the wall of the colon. These pouches can develop when weak spots in the colon's lining bulge outward. When they become infected or irritated, the condition is referred to as diverticulitis. Symptoms include abdominal pain, especially in the lower left side, along with fever, nausea, and changes in bowel habits. A low-fiber diet is often associated with its development. Treatment may involve antibiotics, dietary changes, and, in severe cases, surgical interventions to remove affected segments of the colon. Appropriate handling can aid in symptom relief and avoid problems.

Causes And Risk Factors

Diverticulitis is primarily caused by the formation of small pouches, known as diverticula, in the colon's weak spots. Several factors contribute to the development of diverticulitis, making it essential for beginners to understand the causes and risk factors.

Low-Fiber Diet: A diet low in fiber is a major risk factor. Insufficient fiber intake leads to hard stools, increased colon pressure, and the formation of diverticula.

Aging: As people age, the walls of the colon become weaker, increasing the risk of diverticula formation.

Genetics: Genetics plays a role. If family members have had diverticulitis, you may be at a higher risk.

Obesity: Excess weight, especially around the abdominal area, increases the risk.

Lifestyle: Lack of physical activity and smoking are associated with a higher risk of diverticulitis.

Certain Medications: Long-term use of medications like steroids or nonsteroidal anti-inflammatory drugs can contribute.

Understanding these causes and risk factors is crucial for beginners as it empowers them to make dietary and lifestyle changes that can help prevent or manage diverticulitis effectively. A balanced, high-fiber diet, regular exercise, and other healthy habits can reduce the risk and ease symptoms.

Symptoms And Diagnosis

Diverticulitis can be challenging to understand, especially for beginners. Recognizing the symptoms and the diagnostic process is crucial for early intervention and effective management.

Common Symptoms:

Abdominal Pain: One of the hallmark symptoms is intense, localized pain, usually in the lower left side of the abdomen. It can be sudden and severe.

Fever: If the diverticula becomes infected, it can lead to fever, chills, and an overall feeling of illness.

Change in Bowel Habits: Constipation, diarrhea, or a combination of both can occur.

Nausea and Vomiting: The infection can result in stomach discomfort, nausea, and vomiting.

Bloody Stools: In severe cases, rectal bleeding can happen, leading to bloody stools.

Diagnosis:

To diagnose diverticulitis, healthcare professionals use several methods:

Medical History: They'll discuss your symptoms and medical history to understand your condition better.

Physical Examination: A physical exam to check for tenderness in the abdomen.

Imaging Tests: CT scans are often used to confirm the diagnosis and assess the extent of infection.

Blood Tests: Blood tests can reveal signs of infection and inflammation.

For beginners, recognizing these symptoms and seeking prompt medical attention is crucial. Early diagnosis and treatment can prevent complications and promote a healthy, diverticulitis-free lifestyle.

Diverticulitis Complications

Understanding diverticulitis complications is essential for beginners, as it underscores the importance of early diagnosis and proper management. If left untreated or unmanaged, diverticulitis can lead to several severe complications:

Abscess Formation: Infected diverticula can develop into pockets of pus or abscesses in the abdomen. These abscesses require drainage and antibiotics to resolve.

Perforation: Severe inflammation can cause a diverticulum to rupture, resulting in a perforation of the intestinal wall. This can lead to peritonitis, a life-threatening infection of the abdominal cavity.

Obstruction: Scarring from recurrent inflammation may narrow the colon, causing a partial or complete bowel obstruction. This leads to cramping, bloating, and constipation.

Fistula Formation: In some cases, the inflammation can cause abnormal connections (fistulas) between the colon and nearby structures like the bladder or other parts of the intestine.

These complications emphasize the importance of managing diverticulitis through dietary changes, medication, and, in some cases, surgical intervention. For beginners, early detection and adherence to a diverticulitis-friendly lifestyle can help prevent these serious issues and maintain a good quality of life.

How Diet Affects Diverticulitis

Diet plays a pivotal role in the management of diverticulitis, and understanding how it affects the condition is essential for beginners. In diverticulitis, small pouches or diverticula in the colon become inflamed, often due to trapped stool or bacteria. Diet impacts the condition in several ways:

Fiber Intake: A high-fiber diet is key for diverticulitis management. Fiber keeps stools soft, reducing the risk of inflammation. Beginners should consume ample fruits, vegetables, whole grains, and legumes to maintain regular bowel movements.

Hydration: Staying adequately hydrated is crucial. Water helps prevent constipation, which can exacerbate diverticulitis symptoms.

Foods to Avoid: Certain foods may irritate diverticula or worsen symptoms, including nuts, seeds, and corn. It's often recommended to limit these items, particularly during acute episodes.

Moderation: Proper portion control helps prevent overloading the digestive system, which can trigger diverticulitis flare-ups.

Probiotics: Probiotic-rich foods like yogurt can support a healthy gut microbiome, aiding in overall digestive health.

Beginners should work with healthcare providers and dietitians to develop a personalized diverticulitis-friendly diet plan. A balanced, high-fiber, and well-hydrated diet is often the cornerstone of managing diverticulitis, promoting symptom relief, and reducing the risk of complications.

CHAPTER TWO

MEAL PREP BASICS

Why Meal Prep?

Meal prepping is a valuable practice for beginners dealing with diverticulitis. This condition requires careful dietary management, making meal prepping a logical and effective choice for several reasons:

Controlled Ingredients: By preparing your meals, you have full control over the ingredients, ensuring they align with your diverticulitis-friendly diet. This prevents unwanted surprises or irritants in your food.

Portion Management: Diverticulitis often responds well to well-portioned meals.

Meal prepping allows you to measure and control your portions, reducing the risk of overeating or consuming foods that may trigger symptoms.

Consistency: Regular meals and snacks help regulate bowel movements and keep the digestive system on a steady schedule. Meal prepping ensures you have structured, diverticulitis-friendly meals at hand.

Reduced Stress: The stress of daily meal planning and preparation can be overwhelming, exacerbating diverticulitis symptoms. Meal prepping eases this burden, promoting a more relaxed and stress-free approach to eating.

Time Efficiency: Preparing meals in advance saves time and energy during busy days, reducing the temptation to opt for fast food or less healthy choices.

For beginners, meal prepping isn't just about convenience; it's a proactive strategy for managing diverticulitis effectively. It empowers individuals to maintain a balanced diet, control their intake, and minimize dietary triggers, promoting better symptom management and overall well-being.

Common Mistakes to Avoid While Meal Prepping

Meal prepping is a fantastic strategy for beginners managing diverticulitis, but it's essential to avoid common mistakes to maximize its effectiveness and prevent potential issues:

Lack of Variety: Repetitive meals can become boring, making it more challenging to stick to the plan. Ensure your meal prep includes a variety of foods to keep your diet interesting.

Overcooking: Overcooked foods may lose their nutritional value and become unappetizing. Properly time your cooking to maintain flavor and nutrients.

Poor Storage: Improper storage can lead to food spoilage or contamination. Invest in high-quality, airtight containers to keep your prepped meals fresh and safe.

Ignoring Fiber: A diverticulitis-friendly diet often requires a balance of soluble and insoluble fiber. Don't skip the fiber-rich foods like whole grains, fruits, and vegetables.

Ignoring Medical Advice: It's crucial to consult with a healthcare professional or dietitian when developing your meal prep plan. Ignoring their guidance may lead to a diet that doesn't address your specific diverticulitis needs.

Overlooking Portion Control: Eating too much can cause stomach distress, even when the food is healthful. Eat in moderation, particularly when it comes to heavy or high-fiber foods.

Meal prepping for diverticulitis is a smart approach, but avoiding these mistakes is essential for success.

Portion Control and Monitoring

Portion control and monitoring are essential practices for beginners managing diverticulitis. Controlling the amount of food you consume can help prevent flare-ups and alleviate symptoms. Here are some guidelines:

Balanced Meals: Focus on creating balanced meals that include lean proteins, fiber-rich foods, and healthy fats. Properly portioned meals can provide essential nutrients while preventing excessive strain on the digestive system.

Fiber Awareness: Pay attention to fiber intake. High-fiber foods are important, but excessive fiber at once can be problematic.

Gradually increase your fiber intake and spread it throughout the day.

Regular Meals: Eating regular, small meals rather than a few large ones can help maintain stable blood sugar levels and prevent excessive pressure on the colon.

Hydration: Stay adequately hydrated. Proper fluid intake can help ensure that fiber moves through the digestive tract smoothly, reducing the risk of diverticulitis-related complications.

Listen to Your Body: Be Aware of Signals of Fullness and Hunger. You can learn to identify fullness and prevent overindulgence by eating slowly and deliberately.

Keep a Food Diary: Tracking your meals and symptoms can help identify potential triggers or patterns.

This information is valuable for fine-tuning your portion sizes and food choices. Customizing your portions to suit your individual needs and staying mindful of your body's signals can contribute to better digestive health and a reduced risk of flare-ups.

CHAPTER THREE

Diverticulitis Meal Prep Foods

How to Shop for Diverticulitis Ingredients

Shopping for diverticulitis-friendly ingredients is crucial for maintaining a balanced and digestive-healthy diet. Here are some tips for shopping with diverticulitis in mind:

Focus on Fresh Produce: Opt for fresh fruits and vegetables like apples, pears, carrots, and leafy greens. Fresh produce provides essential vitamins, minerals, and dietary fiber that are gentle on the digestive system.

Choose Lean Proteins: Select lean sources of protein such as poultry, fish, and lean cuts of beef. These options are easier to digest and less likely to irritate the colon.

Whole Grains: Look for whole grains like brown rice, whole wheat pasta, and oats. These grains are rich in fiber and can be a healthy addition to your diet when introduced gradually.

Low-Fat Dairy: Opt for low-fat or fat-free dairy products like yogurt, milk, and cheese. These can provide calcium and protein without excessive saturated fats.

Canned Foods: Choose low-sodium or no-salt-added canned goods to minimize sodium intake, which can lead to water retention and increased pressure on the colon.

Limit Processed Foods: Minimize processed and packaged foods, as they often contain additives and preservatives that may be problematic for individuals with diverticulitis.

Read Labels: Pay attention to food labels, looking for items that are high in fiber but free from seeds or small particles that can be harsh on the digestive tract.

Shopping List Planning: Plan your shopping list in advance, incorporating a variety of ingredients and portion-appropriate foods.

By following these guidelines, you can make informed choices while shopping for diverticulitis-friendly ingredients, helping to maintain a balanced diet that supports digestive health.

Foods to Eat on a Diverticulitis Diet

A diverticulitis diet primarily focuses on consuming foods that are gentle on the digestive system to prevent irritation and inflammation of the diverticula, which are small pouches that can develop in the colon. The key foods to eat on a diverticulitis diet include:

Lean Proteins: Opt for lean sources of protein such as poultry, fish, tofu, and eggs to support muscle health and tissue repair.

Healthy Fats: Include sources of healthy fats like avocados, olive oil, and nuts to maintain overall well-being.

Probiotic Foods: Foods like yogurt and kefir can support a balanced gut microbiome.

Low-Fiber Foods: During a diverticulitis flare-up, a temporary switch to low-fiber foods like white rice, pasta, and well-cooked vegetables can reduce irritation.

It's crucial to remember that the key to managing diverticulitis is to maintain a balanced, high-fiber diet while ensuring that certain foods are minimized during flare-ups.

Foods to Avoid on a Diverticulitis Diet

When managing diverticulitis, it's essential to avoid foods that can irritate or inflame the diverticula, as well as those that might cause digestive discomfort. Here are the foods to steer clear of on a diverticulitis diet:

Nuts and Seeds: These small and hard-to-digest items can get trapped in diverticula and lead to inflammation. It's wise to exclude them from the diet.

Popcorn: The hard shells of popcorn kernels can be problematic, potentially causing irritation or getting lodged in the diverticula.

Spicy Foods: Spices and spicy foods can be irritating to the digestive system and may worsen symptoms during flare-ups.
Red Meat: Red meats can be tough to digest and may not be well-tolerated during diverticulitis episodes. Lean meats like poultry or fish are better options.

Processed Foods: Highly processed foods often contain additives and preservatives that can exacerbate digestive issues. These should be limited.

Sugary Beverages: Excessive sugar can lead to imbalances in the gut microbiome, so it's best to avoid sugary drinks and opt for water or herbal teas instead.

It's important to note that these dietary restrictions may be temporary during acute diverticulitis episodes. Consult with a healthcare professional or registered dietitian for guidance tailored to your specific needs and the stage of your condition.

Low-fiber Foods for Diverticulitis

During diverticulitis flare-ups or in the initial stages of the condition, a low-fiber diet is often recommended. Low-fiber foods are easier on the digestive system and can help reduce irritation and discomfort. These foods may include:

Refined Grains: White bread, pasta, and rice are easier to digest than whole grains. Cooked Fruits and Vegetables: Peeled, well-cooked, and canned varieties can be gentler on the gut.

Lean Proteins: Skinless poultry, fish, and tender cuts of meat are good protein sources.

Dairy: Low-fat dairy products like yogurt and milk are typically well-tolerated.

Eggs: Eggs, especially when prepared without added fats, are a suitable protein option.

Smooth Nut Butter: Creamy, smooth nut butters, such as peanut or almond butter, can be easier to digest.

It's essential to reintroduce high-fiber foods gradually as symptoms subside, as a long-term low-fiber diet is generally discouraged.

High-fiber Foods For Diverticulitis

A high-fiber diet is a cornerstone of managing diverticulitis and promoting digestive health. Foods rich in fiber can help prevent diverticula formation and support regular bowel movements. Examples of high-fiber foods suitable for diverticulitis include:

Whole Grains: Brown rice, whole-grain pasta, and quinoa provide ample fiber.

Fresh Fruits and Vegetables: Berries, apples, spinach, and broccoli are fiber-packed choices.

Legumes: Lentils, chickpeas, and beans offer plant-based protein and fiber.

Nuts and Seeds: Almonds, chia seeds, and flaxseeds are excellent sources of fiber.

Oats: Oatmeal and oat bran are well-tolerated fiber options.

Incorporating these high-fiber foods into your diet can help maintain bowel regularity and reduce the risk of diverticulitis complications. However, it's crucial to drink plenty of water and introduce fiber gradually, especially if you're transitioning from a low-fiber diet.

CHAPTER RECIPES

BREAKFAST RECIPES

Apricot Honey Oatmeal

Serving size: 1

Cooking time: 10 minutes

Ingredients:

- 1/2 cup rolled oats
- 1 cup water
- 1/4 cup dried apricots, chopped
- 1 tablespoon honey
- 1/4 teaspoon cinnamon

Preparation:

1. In a small saucepan, bring the water to a boil.

2. Add the oats and apricots, reduce heat to low, and simmer for 5 minutes.

3. Stir in the honey and cinnamon and cook for an additional 2-3 minutes.

Nutritional value:

270 calories,

4g fat,

57g carbohydrates,

6g fiber,

7g protein

Apple Raisin Pancakes

Serving size: 1

Cooking time: 20 minutes

Ingredients:

- 1/2 cup whole wheat flour
- 1/2 teaspoon baking powder
- 1/4 teaspoon baking soda

•1/4 teaspoon cinnamon

•1/4 cup unsweetened applesauce

•1/4 cup low-fat milk

•1 egg

•1/4 cup raisins

Preparation:

1. In a medium bowl, whisk together the flour, baking powder, baking soda, and cinnamon.

2. In a separate bowl, whisk together the applesauce, milk, and egg.

3. Add the wet ingredients to the dry ingredients and stir until just combined.

4. Fold in the raisins.

5. Heat a nonstick skillet over medium heat and spray with cooking spray.

6. Pour 1/4 cup of batter onto the skillet and cook until bubbles form on the surface, then

7. flip and cook until golden brown.

Nutritional value:

280 calories

4g fat

53g carbohydrates

6g fiber

10g protein

Bran Muffins

Serving size: 1 muffin

Cooking time: 25 minutes

Ingredients:

- 1 cup wheat bran
- 1/2 cup whole wheat flour
- 1/2 teaspoon baking soda
- 1/4 teaspoon salt

•1/4 cup unsweetened applesauce

•1/4 cup honey

•1 egg

•1/2 cup low-fat milk

Preparation:

1. Preheat the oven to 375°F and line a muffin tin with paper liners.

2. In a medium bowl, whisk together the wheat bran, flour, baking soda, and salt.

3. In a separate bowl, whisk together the applesauce, honey, egg, and milk.

4. Add the wet ingredients to the dry ingredients and stir until just combined.

5. Evenly distribute the batter into each muffin cup.

6. Bake for 20-25 minutes, or until a toothpick inserted into the center of a muffin comes out clean.

Nutritional value:

120 calories

1g fat

28g carbohydrates

6g fiber

4g protein

Spinach and Feta Breakfast Wrap

Serving size: 1
Cooking time: 10 minutes

Ingredients:

•1 whole wheat tortilla

•1 egg

•1/4 cup frozen spinach, thawed and drained

•1 tablespoon crumbled feta cheese

Preparation:

1. In a small bowl, whisk together the egg and spinach.

2. Heat a nonstick skillet over medium heat and spray with cooking spray.

3. Pour the egg mixture into the skillet and cook until set, flipping once.

4. Place the egg on the tortilla and sprinkle with feta cheese.

5. Roll up the tortilla and serve.

Nutritional value:
220 calories
9g fat
22g carbohydrates
6g fiber

14g protein

Protein Smoothie

Serving size: 1
Cooking time: 5 minutes

Ingredients:
- 1/2 cup low-fat milk
- 1/2 cup plain Greek yogurt
- 1/2 banana
- 1/2 cup frozen mixed berries
- 1 scoop vanilla protein powder

Preparation:

1. Combine all ingredients in a blender and blend until smooth.

2. Serve immediately.

Nutritional value:

280 calories

3g fat

35g carbohydrates

6g fiber

29g protein

Quinoa and Blueberry Muffins

Serving size: 1 muffin

Cooking time: 25 minutes

Ingredients:

- 1 cup cooked quinoa
- 1/2 cup whole wheat flour
- 1/2 teaspoon baking powder
- 1/4 teaspoon baking soda
- 1/4 teaspoon salt
- 1/4 cup unsweetened applesauce
- 1/4 cup honey
- 1 egg
- 1/2 cup low-fat milk
- 1/2 cup blueberries

Preparation:

1. Preheat the oven to 375°F and line a muffin tin with paper liners.

2. In a medium bowl, whisk together the quinoa, flour, baking powder, baking soda, and salt.

3. In a separate bowl, whisk together the applesauce, honey, egg, and milk.

4. Add the wet ingredients to the dry ingredients and stir until just combined.

5. Fold in the blueberries.

6. Evenly distribute the batter into each muffin cup.

7. Bake for 20-25 minutes, or until a toothpick inserted into the center of a muffin comes out clean.

Nutritional value:

180 calories

2g fat

35g carbohydrates

4g fiber

6g protein

Cranberry Juice

Serving size: 1 cup
Cooking time: 0 minutes

Ingredients:

•1 cup unsweetened cranberry juice

Preparation:

1. Pour the cranberry juice into a glass.

2. Serve chilled.

Nutritional value:

45 calories

0g fat

12g carbohydrates

0g fiber

0g protein

Breakfast Carrot Cake

Serving: 1 slice

Cooking Time: 40 minutes

Ingredients:

•1/2 cup quinoa flour

•1/4 cup grated carrots

•1/4 cup unsweetened applesauce

•2 tablespoons chopped walnuts

•2 tablespoons honey

•1/2 teaspoon baking powder

•1/4 teaspoon cinnamon

•A pinch of salt

Preparation:

1. Preheat the oven to 350°F (175°C) and grease a small baking dish.

2. In a mixing bowl, combine quinoa flour, grated carrots, chopped walnuts, baking powder, cinnamon, and a pinch of salt.

3. In a separate bowl, mix unsweetened applesauce and honey.

4. Combine the wet and dry ingredients and stir until well incorporated.

5. Pour the batter into the prepared baking dish.

6. Bake for about 30-35 minutes or until a toothpick comes out clean when inserted into the cake.

7. Allow it to cool, then slice and serve.

CHAPTER FIVE

LUNCH RECIPES

Grilled Chicken and Brown Rice Bowl

Serving size: 1

Cooking time: 30 minutes

Ingredients:

•4 ounces boneless, skinless chicken breast

•1/2 cup cooked brown rice

•1/2 cup steamed broccoli

•1/4 cup sliced almonds

•1 tablespoon olive oil

•1 tablespoon lemon juice

•1/4 teaspoon salt

•1/4 teaspoon black pepper

Preparation:

1. Heat a grill or grill pan to a medium-high temperature.

2. Sprinkle salt and pepper on the chicken breast.

3. Grill the chicken for 5-6 minutes per side, or until cooked through.

4. In a small bowl, whisk together the olive oil, lemon juice, salt, and pepper.

5. In a serving bowl, combine the cooked brown rice, steamed broccoli, and sliced almonds.

6. Slice the grilled chicken and add it to the bowl.

7. Drizzle the dressing over the top and serve.

Nutritional value:

400 calories

18g fat

28g carbohydrates

6g fiber

32g protein

Tuna and Cucumber Wraps

Serving size: 1

Cooking time: 10 minutes

Ingredients:

- 1 whole wheat tortilla
- 1 can (5 ounces) low-sodium tuna, drained
- 1/4 cup plain Greek yogurt
- 1/4 cup chopped cucumber
- 1/4 teaspoon dried dill

Preparation:

1. In a small bowl, combine the tuna, Greek yogurt, cucumber, and dill.

2. Heat the tortilla in the microwave for 10-15 seconds to soften.

3. Spread the tuna mixture onto the tortilla. Roll up the tortilla and serve.

Nutritional value:
250 calories
5g fat
25g carbohydrates
6g fiber
26g protein

Cilantro Bean Salad

Serving size: 1
Cooking time: 10 minutes

Ingredients:

•1 can (15 ounces) low-sodium black beans, drained and rinsed

•1 can (15 ounces) low-sodium kidney beans, drained and rinsed

•1/2 cup chopped red onion

•1/4 cup chopped fresh cilantro

•2 tablespoons olive oil

•1 tablespoon lime juice

•1/4 teaspoon salt

•1/4 teaspoon black pepper

Preparation:

1. In a medium bowl, combine the black beans, kidney beans, red onion, and cilantro.

2. In a small bowl, whisk together the olive oil, lime juice, salt, and pepper.

3. Drizzle the bean mixture with the dressing and mix thoroughly.

Nutritional value:

280 calories

10g fat

35g carbohydrates

12g fiber

12g protein

Turkey and Cranberry Spinach Salad

Serving size: 1

Cooking time: 10 minutes

Ingredients:

- 2 cups baby spinach
- 4 ounces sliced turkey breast
- 1/4 cup dried cranberries
- 1/4 cup chopped walnuts
- 1 tablespoon olive oil
- 1 tablespoon balsamic vinegar
- 1/4 teaspoon salt
- 1/4 teaspoon black pepper

Preparation:

1. In a large bowl, combine the baby spinach, turkey breast, dried cranberries, and chopped walnuts.

2. In a small bowl, whisk together the olive oil, balsamic vinegar, salt, and pepper.

3. Drizzle the bean mixture with the dressing and mix thoroughly.

Nutritional value:
350 calories
22g fat
18g carbohydrates
4g fiber
22g protein

Garbanzo and Tomato Salad

Serving size: 1

Cooking time: 10 minutes

Ingredients:

•1 can (15 ounces) low-sodium garbanzo beans, drained and rinsed

•1 cup cherry tomatoes, halved

•1/4 cup chopped red onion

•1/4 cup chopped fresh parsley

•2 tablespoons olive oil

•1 tablespoon red wine vinegar

•1/4 teaspoon salt

•1/4 teaspoon black pepper

Preparation:

1. In a medium bowl, combine the garbanzo beans, cherry tomatoes, red onion, and parsley.

2. In a small bowl, whisk together the olive oil, red wine vinegar, salt, and pepper.

3. Drizzle the bean mixture with the dressing and mix thoroughly.

Nutritional value:

280 calories

12g fat

32g carbohydrates

10g fiber

10g protein

Chicken Pasta Salad

Serving size: 1

Cooking time: 20 minutes

Ingredients:

•2 ounces whole wheat pasta

•2 ounces cooked chicken breast, chopped

•1/4 cup chopped cucumber

•1/4 cup chopped red bell pepper

•1/4 cup chopped red onion

•2 tablespoons olive oil

•1 tablespoon red wine vinegar

•1/4 teaspoon salt

•1/4 teaspoon black pepper

Preparation:

1. Cook the pasta according to package instructions.

2. In a large bowl, combine the cooked pasta, chicken breast, cucumber, red bell pepper, and red onion.

3. In a small bowl, whisk together the olive oil, red wine vinegar, salt, and pepper.

4. Drizzle the bean mixture with the dressing and mix thoroughly.

Nutritional value:

350 calories

16g fat

25g carbohydrates

4g fiber

25g protein

Zucchini Noodles with Pesto

Serving size: 1

Cooking time: 15 minutes

Ingredients:

1 medium zucchini, spiralized

1/4 cup prepared pesto

1/4 cup cherry tomatoes, halved

1/4 cup chopped walnuts

Preparation:

1. In a large bowl, combine the spiralized zucchini, pesto, cherry tomatoes, and

chopped walnuts.

2. Toss to combine.

Nutritional value:

300 calories

28g fat

8g carbohydrates

2g fiber

6g protein

Spinach and Mushroom Quiche

Serving size: 1 slice

Cooking time: 45 minutes

Ingredients:

• 1 whole wheat pie crust

• 1 tablespoon olive oil

• 1 onion, chopped

• 2 cloves garlic, minced

• 2 cups baby spinach

- 1 cup sliced mushrooms
- 4 eggs
- 1/2 cup low-fat milk
- 1/4 teaspoon salt
- 1/4 teaspoon black pepper

Preparation:

1. Preheat the oven to 375°F.

2. In a large skillet, heat the olive oil over medium heat.

3. Add the onion and garlic and cook until softened about 5 minutes.

4. Add the spinach and mushrooms and cook until the spinach is wilted and the mushrooms are tender about 5 minutes.

5. In a medium bowl, whisk together the eggs, low-fat milk, salt, and pepper.

6. Spread the spinach and mushroom mixture into the pie crust.

7. Pour the egg mixture over the top.

8. Bake for 30-35 minutes, or until the quiche is set and golden brown.

Nutritional value:
280 calories
18g fat
18g carbohydrates
3g fiber
11g protein

CHAPTER SIX

DINNER RECIPES

Rhubarb Compote

Serving size: 1

Cooking time: 30 minutes

Ingredients:
- 2 cups chopped rhubarb
- 1/4 cup honey
- 1/4 cup water
- 1/2 teaspoon vanilla extract

Preparation:

1. In a medium saucepan, combine the rhubarb, honey, and water.

2. Bring to a boil, then reduce heat and simmer for 20-25 minutes, or until the rhubarb is soft and the mixture has thickened.

3. Stir in the vanilla extract.

4. Serve warm or chilled.

Nutritional value:

120 calories

0g fat

32g carbohydrates

2g fiber

1g protein

Turkey and Sweet Potato Hash

Serving size: 1

Cooking time: 30 minutes

Ingredients:

•4 ounces ground turkey

•1 small sweet potato, peeled and diced

•1/4 cup chopped onion

•1/4 cup chopped red bell pepper

•1/4 teaspoon dried thyme

•1/4 teaspoon salt

•1/4 teaspoon black pepper

Preparation:

1. In a large skillet, cook the ground turkey over medium heat until browned, breaking it up into small pieces.

2. Add the sweet potato, onion, red bell pepper, thyme, salt, and pepper.

3. Cook, stirring occasionally, for 15-20 minutes, or until the sweet potato is tender.

Nutritional value:

250 calories

8g fat

22g carbohydrates

4g fiber

22g protein

Potato and Arugula Salad

Serving size: 1
Cooking time: 30 minutes

Ingredients:

•1 medium potato, peeled and diced

•1/4 cup chopped red onion

•1/4 cup chopped fresh parsley

•2 tablespoons olive oil

•1 tablespoon red wine vinegar

•1/4 teaspoon salt

•1/4 teaspoon black pepper

•2 cups arugula

Preparation:

1. In a medium saucepan, cover the diced potato with water and bring to a boil.

2. Reduce heat and simmer for 10-15 minutes, or until the potato is tender.

3. Drain the potato and let it cool.

4. In a large bowl, combine the cooled potato, red onion, and parsley.

5. In a small bowl, whisk together the olive oil, red wine vinegar, salt, and pepper.

6. Pour the dressing over the potato mixture and toss to combine.

7. Add the arugula and toss again.

Nutritional value:

280 calories

14g fat

32g carbohydrates

6g fiber

6g protein

Cod Fillet with Garlic and Herbs

Serving size: 1
Cooking time: 20 minutes

Ingredients:

•4 ounces cod fillet

•1 tablespoon olive oil

•1 clove garlic, minced

•1/4 teaspoon dried thyme

•1/4 teaspoon salt

•1/4 teaspoon black pepper

Preparation:

1. Preheat the oven to 375°F.

2. In a small bowl, combine the olive oil, garlic, thyme, salt, and pepper.

3. Place the cod fillet on a baking sheet.

5. Brush the olive oil mixture over the top of the cod.

6. Bake for 15-20 minutes, or until the cod is cooked through.

Nutritional value:

150 calories

7g fat

0g carbohydrates

0g fiber

20g protein

Butternut Squash and Quinoa Bake

Serving size: 1

Cooking time: 45 minutes

Ingredients:

- 1 cup cooked quinoa
- 1 cup cubed butternut squash
- 1/4 cup chopped onion
- 1/4 cup chopped red bell pepper
- 1/4 cup chopped fresh parsley
- 2 tablespoons olive oil
- 1 tablespoon balsamic vinegar
- 1/4 teaspoon salt
- 1/4 teaspoon black pepper

Preparation:

1. Preheat the oven to 375°F.

2. In a large bowl, combine the cooked quinoa, butternut squash, onion, red bell pepper, and parsley.

3. In a small bowl, whisk together the olive oil, balsamic vinegar, salt, and pepper.

4. Pour the dressing over the quinoa mixture and toss to combine.

5. Pour the blend into a baking tray.

6. Bake for 25-30 minutes, or until the butternut squash is tender.

Nutritional value:
350 calories
16g fat
45g carbohydrates
8g fiber
8g protein

Provence-Style Cod Casserole

Serving size: 1

Cooking time: 45 minutes

Ingredients:

•4 ounces cod fillet

•1/2 cup chopped onion

•1/2 cup chopped red bell pepper

•1/2 cup chopped zucchini

•1/2 cup chopped eggplant

•1/4 cup chopped fresh parsley

•2 tablespoons olive oil

•1 tablespoon tomato paste

•1/4 teaspoon dried thyme

•1/4 teaspoon salt

•1/4 teaspoon black pepper

Preparation

1. Preheat the oven to 375°F.

2. In a large skillet, heat the olive oil over medium heat.

3. Add the onion, red bell pepper, zucchini, and eggplant.

4. Cook, stirring occasionally, for 10-15 minutes, or until the vegetables are tender.

5. Stir in the tomato paste, thyme, salt, and pepper.

6. Transfer the vegetable mixture to a baking dish.

7. Place the cod fillet on top of the vegetables.

8. Bake for 20-25 minutes, or until the cod is cooked through.

Nutritional value:

300 calories

14g fat

18g carbohydrates

5g fiber

24g protein

Grilled Portobello Mushrooms with Polenta

Serving size: 1

Cooking time: 30 minutes

Ingredients:

•2 large portobello mushroom caps

•1/2 cup cooked polenta

•1/4 cup chopped fresh parsley

•2 tablespoons olive oil

•1 tablespoon balsamic vinegar

•1/4 teaspoon salt

•1/4 teaspoon black pepper

Preparation:

1. Preheat a grill or grill pan over medium-high heat.

2. Brush the portobello mushroom caps with olive oil.

3. Grill the mushrooms for 5-6 minutes per side, or until tender.

4. In a small bowl, whisk together the olive oil, balsamic vinegar, salt, and pepper.

5. In a serving dish, spoon the cooked polenta.

6. Top with the grilled portobello mushrooms.

7. Drizzle the dressing over the top and sprinkle with chopped parsley.

Nutritional value:

250 calories

16g fat

20g carbohydrates

3g fiber

6g protein

Baked Cod with Mashed Potatoes and Green Beans

Serving size: 1

Cooking time: 45 minutes

Ingredients:

•4 ounces cod fillet

•1 medium potato, peeled and diced

•1/2 cup green beans, trimmed

- •2 tablespoons olive oil
- •1 tablespoon lemon juice
- •1/4 teaspoon dried thyme
- •1/4 teaspoon salt
- •1/4 teaspoon black pepper

Preparation:

1. Preheat the oven to 375°F.

2. Place the diced potato in a medium saucepan and cover with water.

3. Bring to a boil, then reduce heat and simmer for 10-15 minutes, or until the potato is tender.

4. Drain the potato and mash it with a fork or potato masher.

5. Steam the green beans for 5-7 minutes, or until tender.

6. In a small bowl, whisk together the olive oil, lemon juice, thyme, salt, and pepper.

7. Place the cod fillet on a baking sheet.
8. Brush the olive oil mixture over the top of the cod.

9. Bake for 15-20 minutes, or until the cod is cooked through. Serve

Nutritional value:

300 calories

14g fat

22g carbohydrates

4g fiber

22g protein

CHAPTER SEVEN

SIDES

Quinoa and Veggie Medley

Serving size: 1

Cooking time: 30 minutes

Ingredients:

- 1/2 cup cooked quinoa
- 1/4 cup chopped red onion
- 1/4 cup chopped red bell pepper
- 1/4 cup chopped zucchini
- 1/4 cup chopped eggplant
- 1/4 cup chopped fresh parsley
- 2 tablespoons olive oil
- 1 tablespoon balsamic vinegar
- 1/4 teaspoon salt
- 1/4 teaspoon black pepper

Preparation:

1. In a large bowl, combine the cooked quinoa, red onion, red bell pepper, zucchini, eggplant, and parsley.

2. In a small bowl, whisk together the olive oil, balsamic vinegar, salt, and pepper.

3. Pour the dressing over the quinoa mixture and toss to combine.

Nutritional value:

250 calories

14g fat

28g carbohydrates

6g fiber

6g protein

Garlic Butter Asparagus

Serving size: 1

Cooking time: 15 minutes

Ingredients:

•6-8 asparagus spears

•1 tablespoon butter

•1 clove garlic, minced

•1/4 teaspoon salt

•1/4 teaspoon black pepper

Preparation:

1. Preheat the oven to 375°F.

2. Arrange the spears of asparagus on a sheet pan.

3. Melt the butter in a small saucepan over low heat.

4. Add the minced garlic, salt, and pepper to the melted butter and stir to combine.

5. Brush the garlic butter mixture over the asparagus spears.

6. Bake for 10-12 minutes, or until the asparagus is tender.

Nutritional value:

70 calories

6g fat

4g carbohydrates

2g fiber

2g protein

Roasted Asparagus with Lemon Zest

Serving size: 1

Cooking time: 15 minutes

Ingredients:

•6-8 asparagus spears

•1 tablespoon olive oil

•1/2 teaspoon lemon zest

•1/4 teaspoon salt

•1/4 teaspoon black pepper

Preparation:

1. Preheat the oven to 375°F.

2. Place the asparagus spears on a baking sheet.

3. Drizzle the olive oil over the asparagus spears.

4. Sprinkle the lemon zest, salt, and pepper over the top.

5. Bake for 10-12 minutes, or until the asparagus is tender.

Nutritional value:

70 calories

6g fat

4g carbohydrates

2g fiber

2g protein

Mashed Cauliflower with Chives

Serving size: 1

Cooking time: 30 minutes

Ingredients:

- 1/2 head cauliflower, chopped
- 1 tablespoon butter
- 1 tablespoon chopped fresh chives
- 1/4 teaspoon salt
- 1/4 teaspoon black pepper

Preparation:

1. Place the chopped cauliflower in a medium saucepan and cover with water.

2. Bring to a boil, then reduce heat and simmer for 10-15 minutes, or until the cauliflower is tender.

3. Drain the cauliflower and return it to the saucepan.

4. Add the butter, chives, salt, and pepper. Mash the cauliflower with a fork or potato masher until it reaches the desired consistency.

Nutritional value:
70 calories
6g fat
4g carbohydrates
2g fiber
2g protein

Herbed Brown Rice

Serving size: 1
Cooking time: 45 minutes

Ingredients:
- 1/2 cup brown rice
- 1 cup water
- 1 tablespoon chopped fresh parsley
- 1 tablespoon chopped fresh thyme
- 1/4 teaspoon salt
- 1/4 teaspoon black pepper

Preparation:

1. In a medium saucepan, combine the brown rice and water.

2. Bring to a boil, then reduce heat and simmer for 35-40 minutes, or until the rice is tender.

3. Stir in the chopped parsley, thyme, salt, and pepper.

Nutritional value:

120 calories

1g fat

24g carbohydrates

2g fiber

3g protein

Light Shrimp and Barley Salad

Serving size: 1

Cooking time: 30 minutes

Ingredients:

•1/2 cup cooked barley

•4 ounces cooked shrimp

•1/4 cup chopped cucumber

•1/4 cup chopped red bell pepper

•1/4 cup chopped red onion

•2 tablespoons olive oil

•1 tablespoon lemon juice

•1/4 teaspoon salt

•1/4 teaspoon black pepper

Preparation:

1. In a large bowl, combine the cooked barley, cooked shrimp, cucumber, red bell pepper, and red onion.

2. In a small bowl, whisk together the olive oil, lemon juice, salt, and pepper.

3. Pour the dressing over the barley mixture and toss to combine.

Nutritional value:

250 calories

10g fat

22g carbohydrates

4g fiber

18g protein

Baked Artichoke Dip

Serving size: 1

Cooking time: 30 minutes

Ingredients:

- 1 can artichoke hearts, drained and chopped
- 1/2 cup low-fat mayonnaise
- 1/2 cup grated Parmesan cheese
- 1/4 cup chopped green onions
- 1/4 teaspoon garlic powder
- 1/4 teaspoon black pepper

Preparation:

1. Preheat the oven to 375°F.

2. In a medium bowl, combine the chopped artichoke hearts, low-fat mayonnaise, grated Parmesan cheese, chopped green onions, garlic powder, and black pepper.

3. Transfer the mixture to a baking dish.

4. Bake for 20-25 minutes, or until the dip is hot and bubbly.

Nutritional value:

150 calories

10g fat

8g carbohydrates

2g fiber

8g protein

Broccoli and Potato Casserole

Serving size: 1

Cooking time: 45 minutes

Ingredients:

•1 medium potato, peeled and sliced

•1 cup chopped broccoli

•1/4 cup chopped onion

•1/4 cup low-fat milk

•1/4 cup grated Parmesan cheese

•1/4 teaspoon salt

•1/4 teaspoon black pepper

Preparation:

1. Preheat the oven to 375°F.

2. In a medium saucepan, cover the sliced potato with water and bring to a boil.

3. Reduce heat and simmer for 10-15 minutes, or until the potato is tender.

4. Drain the potato and let it cool.

5. In a large bowl, combine the cooled potato, chopped broccoli, chopped onion, low-fat milk, grated Parmesan cheese, salt, and pepper.

6. Spoon mixture into baking dish.

7. Bake for 25-30 minutes, or until the casserole is hot and bubbly.

Nutritional value:
200 calories
6g fat
28g carbohydrates
4g fiber
10g protein

CHAPTER EIGHT

SNACK RECIPES

Homemade Veggie Chips

Serving: 1

Preparation Time: 25 minutes

Cooking Time: 15 minutes

Ingredients:

•1 medium sweet potato, washed and thinly sliced

•1 medium zucchini, washed and thinly sliced

•1 tablespoon olive oil

•1/2 teaspoon salt

•1/4 teaspoon black pepper

•1/4 teaspoon garlic powder

Preparation:

1. Preheat your oven to 375°F (190°C).

2. In a large bowl, toss the sweet potato and zucchini slices with olive oil, salt, pepper, and garlic powder until they are well-coated.

3. Arrange the slices on a baking sheet in a single layer.

4. Bake for about 15 minutes, or until they are crispy and lightly browned.

5. Remove from the oven and let them cool.

Nutritional Value (Approximate):

Calories: 150

Carbohydrates: 22g

Protein: 3g

Fat: 6g

Fiber: 4g

Almond Butter and Banana Rice Cakes

Serving: 1

Preparation Time: 5 minutes

Ingredients:

• 1 rice cake

• 1 tablespoon almond butter (diverticulitis-friendly nut butter)

• 1/2 banana, sliced

Preparation:

1. Spread the almond butter evenly on the rice cake.

2. Arrange the banana slices on top of the almond butter.

Nutritional Value (Approximate):

Calories: 180

Carbohydrates: 24g

Protein: 5g

Fat: 8g

Fiber: 3g

Kidney Bean Salsa

Serving: 1
Cooking Time: 10 minutes

Ingredients:

•1/2 cup canned kidney beans, drained and rinsed

•1/2 cup diced tomatoes

•2 tablespoons finely diced red onion

•2 tablespoons chopped fresh cilantro

•1/2 lime, juiced

•Salt and pepper to taste

Preparation:

1. In a mixing bowl, combine the kidney beans, diced tomatoes, red onion, and fresh cilantro.

2. Squeeze the juice of half a lime over the mixture.

3. Season with a pinch of salt and pepper to taste.

4. Gently toss all the ingredients to combine thoroughly.

5. Serve immediately as a refreshing salsa dip with rice cakes or enjoy it as a topping for whole-grain crackers.

Nutritional Value (Approximate):
Calories: 200
Carbohydrates: 40g

Protein: 10g

Fat: 0.5g

Fiber: 11g

Vitamin C: 12% of daily value

Iron: 10% of daily value

Mini Salmon Cakes with Lemon Aioli

Serving: 1
Cooking Time: 20 minutes

Ingredients:

•4 oz canned salmon, drained

•1/4 cup whole wheat breadcrumbs

•1 egg

•2 tablespoons chopped green onions

•1/2 teaspoon dried dill

•1/2 lemon, juiced

•Salt and pepper to taste

Preparation:

1. In a bowl, combine drained canned salmon, whole wheat breadcrumbs, egg, chopped green onions, dried dill, and the juice of half a lemon.

2. Season the mixture with a pinch of salt and pepper.

3. Mix well until it holds together.

4. Form the mixture into mini patties.

5. In a non-stick pan, heat a small amount of olive oil over medium heat.

6. Cook the salmon cakes until they are golden brown on each side (approximately 3-4 minutes per side).

Nutritional Value (Approximate):

Calories: 300

Carbohydrates: 15g

Protein: 22g

Fat: 16g

Fiber: 2g

Greek Lettuce Wraps

Serving: 1

Preparation Time: 15 minutes

Ingredients:

•2 large lettuce leaves (e.g., Romaine or Iceberg)

•4 oz cooked chicken breast, diced

•1/4 cup diced cucumber

•1/4 cup diced tomatoes

•2 tablespoons crumbled feta cheese

•2 tablespoons plain Greek yogurt

•1/2 teaspoon dried oregano

•Salt and pepper to taste

Preparation:

1. Carefully wash and pat dry the lettuce leaves.

2. In a bowl, combine diced cooked chicken breast, diced cucumber, diced tomatoes, crumbled feta cheese, and dried oregano.

3. Add plain Greek yogurt to the mixture, and season with salt and pepper to taste.

4. Fill each lettuce leaf with the chicken and veggie mixture.

5. Wrap them like tacos and serve.

Nutritional Value (Approximate):
Calories: 350
Carbohydrates: 8g
Protein: 45g
Fat: 14g

Fiber: 2g

Cucumber Dill Bites

Serving: 1
Preparation Time: 10 minutes

Ingredients:
- 1 cucumber, sliced into rounds
- 2 tablespoons plain Greek yogurt
- 1 teaspoon fresh dill, chopped
- Salt and pepper to taste

Preparation:

1. Arrange the cucumber slices on a plate.

2. In a small bowl, mix plain Greek yogurt, fresh dill, salt, and pepper.

3. Place a small dollop of the yogurt-dill mixture on each cucumber round. Serve

Nutritional Value (Approximate):

Calories: 60

Carbohydrates: 9g

Protein: 4g

Fat: 1g

Fiber: 2g

Honey Baked Apples

Serving: 1

Preparation Time: 30 minutes

Ingredients:

•1 small apple, cored and sliced

•1/2 teaspoon honey

•1/2 teaspoon ground cinnamon

•1 teaspoon chopped walnuts (optional)

Preparation:

1. Preheat your oven to 375°F (190°C).

2. In a baking dish, place the apple slices.

3. Drizzle honey over the apple slices and sprinkle them with ground cinnamon.

4. If desired, add chopped walnuts for a crunchy texture.

5. Bake for about 20-25 minutes until the apples are tender and lightly caramelized.

Nutritional Value (Approximate):

Calories: 90

Carbohydrates: 25g

Protein: 0.5g

Fat: 0.5g

Fiber: 4g

Baked Sweet Potato Fries

Serving: 1

Preparation Time: 35 minutes

Ingredients:

•1 medium sweet potato, cut into fries

•1/2 teaspoon olive oil

•1/2 teaspoon paprika

•Salt and pepper to taste

Preparation:

1. Preheat your oven to 425°F (220°C).

2. In a bowl, toss sweet potato fries with olive oil, paprika, salt, and pepper.

3. Arrange the fries on a baking sheet in a single layer.

4. Bake for approximately 25-30 minutes, or until the fries are crispy.

Nutritional Value (Approximate):

Calories: 130

Carbohydrates: 30g

Protein: 2g

Fat: 1g

Fiber: 5g

CHAPTER NINE

SOUP & STEW RECIPES

Beans with Greens Soup

Serving: 1

Preparation Time: 30 minutes

Ingredients:

• 1 cup cooked navy beans

• 1 cup fresh spinach, chopped

• 1/2 cup low-sodium vegetable broth

• 1/4 teaspoon minced garlic

• 1/4 teaspoon dried thyme

• Salt and pepper to taste

Preparation:

1. In a pot, combine the cooked navy beans, chopped fresh spinach, low-sodium

vegetable broth, minced garlic, and dried thyme.

2. Bring the mixture to a simmer and cook for 20 minutes.

3. Season with salt and pepper to taste. Serve hot.

Nutritional Value (Approximate):
Calories: 200
Carbohydrates: 40g
Protein: 15g
Fat: 1g
Fiber: 8g

Potato Leek Soup

Serving: 1
Preparation Time: 35 minutes

Ingredients:

•1 medium potato, peeled and diced

•1/2 leek, sliced

•1 cup low-sodium vegetable broth

•1/4 cup plain Greek yogurt

•1/4 teaspoon dried thyme

•Salt and pepper to taste

Preparation:

1. In a pot, combine the diced potato, sliced leek, low-sodium vegetable broth, and dried thyme.

2. Bring to a simmer and cook for 20-25 minutes until the potato is tender.

3. Blend the soup until smooth.

4. Stir in plain Greek yogurt and season with salt and pepper.

5. Reheat and serve.

Nutritional Value (Approximate):

Calories: 180

Carbohydrates: 35g

Protein: 8g

Fat: 1g

Fiber: 5g

Hearty Vegetable and Barley Stew

Serving: 1
Preparation Time: 45 minutes

Ingredients:

- 1/4 cup barley
- 1/2 cup diced carrots
- 1/2 cup diced zucchini
- 1/2 cup diced celery
- 1/2 cup low-sodium vegetable broth
- 1/4 teaspoon dried thyme

•Salt and pepper to taste

Preparation:

1. In a pot, combine barley, diced carrots, diced zucchini, diced celery, low-sodium vegetable broth, and dried thyme.

2. Bring to a simmer and cook for 30-35 minutes until the barley and veggies are tender.

3. Season with salt and pepper. Serve

Nutritional Value (Approximate):

Calories: 200

Carbohydrates: 45g

Protein: 5g

Fat: 1g

Fiber: 8g

Tomato Basil Bisque

Serving: 1
Preparation Time: 30 minutes

Ingredients:
•1 cup diced tomatoes (canned, no salt added)
•1/2 cup low-sodium vegetable broth
•1/4 cup plain Greek yogurt
•1/4 teaspoon dried basil
•Salt and pepper to taste

Preparation:

1. In a pot, combine diced tomatoes, low-sodium vegetable broth, and dried basil.

2. Bring to a simmer and cook for 20 minutes.

3. Blend the mixture until smooth.

4. Stir in plain Greek yogurt and season with salt and pepper.

5. Reheat and serve.

Nutritional Value (Approximate):

Calories: 100

Carbohydrates: 15g

Protein: 7g

Fat: 1g

Fiber: 3g

Spinach and White Bean Minestrone

Serving: 1

Preparation Time: 40 minutes

Ingredients:

•1/2 cup canned white beans (no salt added)

•1/2 cup chopped fresh spinach

•1/4 cup diced tomatoes (canned, no salt added)
•1/4 cup diced carrots
•1/4 cup diced celery
•1/2 cup low-sodium vegetable broth
•1/4 teaspoon dried oregano
•Salt and pepper to taste

Preparation:

1. In a pot, combine white beans, chopped fresh spinach, diced tomatoes, diced carrots, diced celery, low-sodium vegetable broth, and dried oregano.

2. Bring to a simmer and cook for 30 minutes until the vegetables are tender.

3. Season with salt and pepper. Serve hot.

Nutritional Value (Approximate):

Calories: 180

Carbohydrates: 35g

Protein: 8g

Fat: 1g

Fiber: 8g

Cannellini and Butter Bean Soup

Serving: 1

Preparation Time: 35 minutes

Ingredients:

•1/4 cup canned cannellini beans (no salt added)

•1/4 cup canned butter beans (no salt added)

•1/2 cup low-sodium vegetable broth

•1/4 cup diced zucchini

•1/4 cup diced carrots

•1/4 cup diced celery

•1/4 teaspoon dried rosemary

•Salt and pepper to taste

Preparation:

1. In a pot, combine cannellini beans, butter beans, low-sodium vegetable broth, diced zucchini, diced carrots, diced celery, and dried rosemary.

2. Bring to a simmer and cook for 25-30 minutes until the vegetables are tender.

3. Season with salt and pepper. Serve warm.

Nutritional Value (Approximate):

Calories: 150

Carbohydrates: 30g

Protein: 7g

Fat: 1g

Fiber: 6g

Creamy Mushroom Bisque

Serving: 1

Preparation Time: 30 minutes

Ingredients:
- 1 cup sliced mushrooms
- 1/2 cup low-sodium vegetable broth
- 1/4 cup plain Greek yogurt
- 1/4 teaspoon dried thyme
- Salt and pepper to taste

Preparation:

1. In a pot, combine sliced mushrooms, low-sodium vegetable broth, and dried thyme.

2. Bring to a simmer and cook for 20-25 minutes until the mushrooms are tender.

3. Blend the mixture until smooth.

4. Stir in plain Greek yogurt and season with salt and pepper.

5. Reheat and serve.

Nutritional Value (Approximate):

Calories: 100

Carbohydrates: 10g

Protein: 6g

Fat: 1g

Fiber: 2g

Pea and Ham Soup

Serving: 1

Preparation Time: 35 minutes

Ingredients:

•1/2 cup cooked peas

•1/4 cup diced ham (low-sodium)

•1/2 cup low-sodium vegetable broth

•1/4 cup diced carrots

•1/4 cup diced celery

•1/4 teaspoon dried thyme

•Salt and pepper to taste

Preparation:

1. In a pot, combine cooked peas, diced ham, low-sodium vegetable broth, diced carrots, diced celery, and dried thyme.

2. Bring to a simmer and cook for 25-30 minutes until the vegetables are tender.

3. Season with salt and pepper. Serve hot.

Nutritional Value (Approximate):

Calories: 180

Carbohydrates: 30g

Protein: 15g

Fat: 2g

Fiber: 7g

CHAPTER TEN

DESSERT RECIPES

Cinnamon Raisin Bread Pudding

Serving: 1

Preparation Time: 40 minutes

Ingredients:
- 1/2 cup diced whole grain bread (no crust)
- 1/4 cup raisins
- 1/2 cup skim milk
- 1/4 teaspoon ground cinnamon
- 1/4 teaspoon vanilla extract

Preparation:

1. In a bowl, combine diced whole-grain bread, raisins, skim milk, ground cinnamon, and vanilla extract.

2. Let it sit for 30 minutes to allow the bread to soak up the milk.

3. Preheat the oven to 350°F (175°C).

4. Transfer the mixture to an oven-safe dish.

5. Bake for 25-30 minutes until the top is golden. Serve warm.

Nutritional Value (Approximate):

Calories: 220

Carbohydrates: 46g

Protein: 7g

Fat: 1g

Fiber: 4g

Coconut Macaroons

Serving: 1

Preparation Time: 25 minutes

Ingredients:

- 1/4 cup unsweetened shredded coconut
- 1/4 cup egg whites
- 1/4 teaspoon vanilla extract
- 1 tablespoon honey

Preparation:

1. Preheat the oven to 325°F (160°C).

2. In a bowl, combine unsweetened shredded coconut, egg whites, vanilla extract, and honey.

3. Spoonfuls of the mixture should be dropped onto a baking sheet.

4. Bake for 15-20 minutes until the macaroons are lightly browned.

5. Allow them to cool before serving.

Nutritional Value (Approximate):

Calories: 160

Carbohydrates: 15g

Protein: 3g

Fat: 8g

Fiber: 3g

Fruit Salad

Serving: 1

Preparation Time: 15 minutes

Ingredients:

•1/2 cup diced melon

•1/2 cup diced pineapple

•1/2 cup diced peaches

•1/2 cup seedless grapes

•1 tablespoon honey

Preparation:

1. In a bowl, combine diced melon, diced pineapple, diced peaches, seedless grapes, and honey.

2. Toss the fruits gently until they are well coated. Serve immediately.

Nutritional Value (Approximate):
Calories: 170
Carbohydrates: 44g
Protein: 2g
Fat: 1g
Fiber: 3g

Jello

Serving: 1

Preparation Time: 4 hours (refrigeration time)

Ingredients:
- 1/4 cup sugar-free gelatin (any flavor)
- 1/2 cup boiling water
- 1/2 cup cold water

Preparation:

1. In a bowl, dissolve sugar-free gelatin in boiling water.

2. Stir in cold water.

3. Pour the mixture into a bowl or mold.

4. Refrigerate for at least 4 hours or until set. Serve chilled.

Nutritional Value (Approximate):

Calories: 10

Carbohydrates: 1g

Protein: 2g

Fat: 0g

Sugar: 0g

Lemon Bars

Serving: 1

Preparation Time: 45 minutes

Ingredients:

•1/4 cup whole grain flour

•1/4 cup lemon juice (freshly squeezed)

•1/4 cup honey

•1/4 teaspoon grated lemon zest

•1/4 teaspoon baking powder

•1/4 teaspoon salt

•Powdered sugar (for dusting)

Preparation:

1. Preheat the oven to 350°F (175°C).

2. In a bowl, combine whole grain flour, lemon juice, honey, grated lemon zest, baking powder, and salt.

3. Mix until the batter is smooth.

4. Transfer the batter to a greased baking dish.

5. Bake for 25-30 minutes until the top is golden.

6. Let it cool before dusting with powdered sugar.

7. Cut into bars and serve.

Nutritional Value (Approximate):

Calories: 180

Carbohydrates: 45g

Protein: 3g

Fat: 1g

Fiber: 2g

Oatmeal Cookies

Serving: 1

Preparation Time: 30 minutes

Ingredients:
- 1/4 cup whole grain oats
- 1/4 cup unsweetened applesauce
- 1/4 cup chopped walnuts
- 1/4 teaspoon ground cinnamon
- 1 tablespoon honey

Preparation:

1. Preheat the oven to 350°F (175°C).

2. In a bowl, combine whole-grain oats, unsweetened applesauce, chopped walnuts, ground cinnamon, and honey.

3. Mix well.

4. Spoonfuls of the mixture should be dropped onto a baking sheet.

5. Bake for 15-20 minutes until the cookies are lightly browned.

6. Allow them to cool before serving.

Nutritional Value (Approximate):
Calories: 150
Carbohydrates: 20g
Protein: 3g
Fat: 7g
Fiber: 3g

Peach Cobbler

Serving: 1

Preparation Time: 45 minutes

Ingredients:
- 1/2 cup sliced peaches (canned in juice)
- 1/4 cup whole grain flour
- 1/4 cup rolled oats
- 1/4 cup unsweetened applesauce
- 1/4 teaspoon ground cinnamon
- 1 tablespoon honey

Preparation:

1. Preheat the oven to 350°F (175°C).

2. In a bowl, combine sliced peaches, whole grain flour, rolled oats, unsweetened applesauce, ground cinnamon, and honey.

3. Mix well.

4. Transfer the mixture to an oven-safe dish.

5. Bake for 30-35 minutes until the top is golden and bubbling.

6. Let it cool slightly before serving.

Nutritional Value (Approximate):
Calories: 250
Carbohydrates: 56g
Protein: 4g
Fat: 3g
Fiber: 6g

Rice Pudding

Serving: 1
Preparation Time: 40 minutes

Ingredients:
•1/4 cup white rice
•1 cup skim milk

•1/4 teaspoon ground cinnamon

•1/4 teaspoon vanilla extract

•1 tablespoon honey

Preparation:

1. In a saucepan, combine white rice and skim milk.

2. Bring to a boil, then reduce heat and simmer for 20-25 minutes, stirring occasionally until rice is tender and the mixture thickens.

3. Remove from heat and stir in ground cinnamon, vanilla extract, and honey.

4. Let it cool before serving.

Nutritional Value (Approximate):

Calories: 290

Carbohydrates: 60g

Protein: 8g

Fat: 2g

Strawberry Shortcake

Serving: 1

Preparation Time: 20 minutes

Ingredients:

•1 slice of whole grain angel food cake (store-bought or homemade)

•1/2 cup fresh strawberries, sliced

•1/4 cup low-fat whipped topping

Preparation:

1. Place a slice of whole grain angel food cake on a serving plate.

2. Arrange the sliced fresh strawberries on top of the cake.

3. Add a dollop of low-fat whipped topping over the strawberries.

4. You can garnish with additional fresh strawberries if desired.

Nutritional Value (Approximate):
Calories: 180
Carbohydrates: 40g
Protein: 3g
Fat: 1g
Fiber: 4g

7-DAY MEAL PLAN

Day 1

Breakfast:

Cranberry Juice

Quinoa and Blueberry Muffins

Lunch:

Grilled Chicken and Brown Rice Bowl

Garlic Butter Asparagus

Dinner:

Rhubarb Compote

Potato and Arugula Salad

Day 2

Breakfast:

Apricot Honey Oatmeal

Protein Smoothie

Lunch:

Chicken Pasta Salad

Light Shrimp and Barley Salad

Dinner:

Turkey and Sweet Potato Hash

Baked Artichoke Dip

Day 3

Breakfast:

Bran Muffins

Quinoa and Veggie Medley

Lunch:

Tuna and Cucumber Wraps

Roasted Asparagus with Lemon Zest

Dinner:

Provence-Style Cod Casserole

Herbed Brown Rice

Day 4

Breakfast:

Apple Raisin Pancakes

Spinach and Feta Breakfast Wrap

Lunch:

Zucchini Noodles with Pesto

Broccoli and Potato Casserole

Dinner*:*

Cod Fillet with Garlic and Herbs

Grilled Portobello Mushrooms with Polenta

Day 5

Breakfast*:*

Breakfast Carrot Cake

Almond Butter and Banana Rice Cakes

Lunch*:*

Spinach and Mushroom Quiche

Mashed Cauliflower with Chives

Dinner*:*

Butternut Squash and Quinoa Bake

Mashed Cauliflower with Chives

Day 6

Breakfast*:*

Quinoa and Blueberry Muffins

Bran Muffins

Lunch*:*

Cilantro Bean Salad

Mashed Cauliflower with Chives

Dinner:

Turkey and Cranberry Spinach Salad

Butternut Squash and Quinoa Bake

Day 7

Breakfast:

Protein Smoothie

Bran Muffins

Lunch:

Garbanzo and Tomato Salad

Garlic Butter Asparagus

Dinner:

Potato and Arugula Salad

Grilled Portobello Mushrooms with Polenta

This meal plan provides a variety of recipes to ensure a balanced and nutritious diet for those managing diverticulitis. Enjoy your meals

CONCLUSION

In conclusion, embarking on a diverticulitis meal prep journey for beginners is more than just about managing your health; it's a commitment to a lifestyle that will significantly improve your overall well-being. You've learned the ins and outs of diverticulitis, discovered delicious recipes tailored to your specific dietary needs, and embraced the art of meal preparation. As you reflect on this culinary voyage, remember that your choices in the kitchen play a pivotal role in your health and comfort.

By adopting and adapting to this diverticulitis-friendly diet, you're taking control of your health in a proactive way. You're ensuring that your body receives the nourishment it deserves while reducing the risk of flare-ups and complications related to diverticulitis. The meal prep process empowers you to make thoughtful decisions about the foods you consume, giving you the tools to manage your condition effectively.

Maintaining a diverticular-friendly diet doesn't mean sacrificing flavor or enjoyment. It's about exploring new tastes, textures, and combinations that will delight your palate and satisfy your nutritional needs. As you continue on this path, remember that your journey to a diverticulitis-free life is not only a personal triumph but an inspiration to others who may face similar challenges.

Consistency is the key to a successful meal prep schedule. Stick with the habits you've developed, and let them become an integral part of your life. By staying dedicated to this diverticulitis-friendly diet, you're making a lasting investment in your health, one meal at a time.

So, take this newfound knowledge, embrace these diverticulitis meal prep strategies, and continue this culinary adventure with confidence. Your health and vitality are worth every bite.